FOETAL ALCOHOL SYNDROME

THE RIGHT SUPPORT FOR PATIENTS OF FOETAL ALCOHOL SYNDROME

DR. PERRY DOUGLAS

Contents

CHAPTER ONE

INTRODUCTION

Fetal alcohol syndrome is a circumstance in a little one that outcomes from alcohol publicity for the duration of the mother's pregnancy. Fetal alcohol syndrome causes mind harm and increase problems. The issues due to fetal alcohol syndrome range from little one to infant, however defects as a result of fetal alcohol syndrome aren't reversible.

There may be no amount of alcohol that is recounted to be safe to devour at some point of pregnancy. In case you drink at some point of pregnancy, you location your baby at risk of fetal alcohol syndrome.

If you suspect your little one has fetal alcohol syndrome, communicate to your doctor as speedy as possible. Early prognosis might also assist to lessen troubles inclusive of studying problems and behavioral issues.

A permanent situation, fetal alcohol syndrome (FAS) occurs at the same time as someone consumes any quantity of alcohol for the duration of a being pregnant. Alcohol use all through being pregnant can intrude with the child's development, inflicting physical and intellectual defects. Fetal alcohol syndrome is the most extreme circumstance inside a set of situations called fetal alcohol spectrum problems (FASDs).

Fetal alcohol syndrome (FAS) is a

circumstance that develops in a fetus (growing toddler) while a pregnant man or woman drinks alcohol within the direction of being pregnant. A syndrome is a group of signs and symptoms that occur collectively as the end end result of a specific disease or odd situation. Whilst someone has fetal alcohol syndrome, they're on the most extreme quit of what are known as fetal alcohol spectrum troubles (FASDs).

FAS is a life-lengthy condition which can't be cured. This situation may be avoided if you don't drink any alcohol inside the path of pregnancy. It's possible that even small portions of alcohol consumed in the course of being pregnant can damage your developing fetus.

Fetal alcohol syndrome is the maximum intense fetal alcohol spectrum disease. These are a fixed of start defects that could happen even as a pregnant woman beverages alcohol. Exclusive fetal alcohol syndrome troubles (FASDs) encompass:

Partial fetal alcohol syndrome

Alcohol-related shipping defects

Alcohol-related neurodevelopment disorder

Neurobehavioral disorder associated with prenatal alcohol exposure

Signs

The severity of fetal alcohol syndrome symptoms and signs and symptoms varies, with some children experiencing them to a far extra degree than others. Signs and symptoms and signs and symptoms of fetal alcohol syndrome can also consist of any mix of physical defects, intellectual or cognitive disabilities, and issues functioning and managing each day lifestyles.

Physical defects

Physical defects can also encompass:

Precise facial talents, such as small eyes, a really thin pinnacle lip, a quick, upturned nose, and a easy pores and skin floor most of the nostril and pinnacle lip

Deformities of joints, limbs and fingers

Slow physical increase earlier than and after delivery

Vision issues or hearing troubles

Small head circumference and brain length

Coronary heart defects and troubles with kidneys and bones

Mind and significant nervous system problems

Troubles with the brain and critical worried system may additionally additionally encompass:

Horrific coordination or balance

Intellectual incapacity, gaining knowledge of problems and delayed development

Horrific memory

Hassle with interest and with processing information

Hassle with reasoning and problem-solving

Trouble identifying consequences of picks

Terrible judgment abilties

Jitteriness or hyperactivity

Abruptly changing moods

Social and behavioral problems

Problems in functioning, coping and interacting with others may also encompass:

Hassle in school

Trouble getting together with others

Negative social talents

Problem adapting to alternate or switching from one undertaking to any other

Issues with behavior and impulse control

Bad idea of time

Troubles staying on project

Problem making plans or running towards a aim

Even as a fetus is exposed to alcohol in advance than starting, the little one's development may be affected in plenty of various procedures. The effect of alcohol use may additionally create moderate or immoderate signs. Fetal alcohol spectrum sickness (FASD) is that this organisation of signs and symptoms and signs and symptoms on a scale from least to most consequences. Fetal alcohol syndrome is the maximum intense condition in this scale. Other conditions below the FASD umbrella embody:

Partial fetal alcohol syndrome (pFAS): people with pFAS have some of the traits of FAS (adjustments to their facial competencies, for instance), but don't have all of the symptoms and signs and symptoms for FAS.

Alcohol-related neurodevelopmental disorder (ARND): people with this disease revel in some or all of the following: impulsiveness, inattentiveness and challenges with judgment and college ordinary overall performance.

Alcohol-related delivery defects (ARBD): the ones are bodily beginning defects (unusual modifications to components of the frame) that could have an effect on the coronary heart, eyes, skeletal gadget, ears and kidneys.

Neurobehavioral ailment associated with prenatal alcohol exposure (ND-PAE): a person with this circumstance come to be exposed to more than a small quantity of alcohol as a fetus. They've got problem with daily duties like bathing and might warfare in social settings because of huge behavior issues like excessive tantrums. Similarly they have problem with wondering and memory.

CHAPTER TWO

What reasons fetal alcohol syndrome (FAS)?

Fetal alcohol syndrome happens while someone beverages any alcohol at some point of being pregnant, together with wine, beer, hard ciders and "tough liquor". Without alcohol use, FAS doesn't occur. One cause alcohol is volatile within the direction of pregnancy is that it's handed via your bloodstream to the fetus through the umbilical wire. The infant doesn't metabolize (destroy down) alcohol inside the same manner an adult does – it remains in the body for an prolonged time body.

Alcohol can intervene with the ordinary

development of the fetus, particularly the mind and crucial involved device. This takes place in any of the subsequent tactics:

Alcohol can kill cells in distinct elements of the fetus, inflicting strange physical development.

Alcohol interferes with the manner nerve cells expand, how they tour to shape wonderful components of the mind and their functioning.

Alcohol constricts blood vessels, which slows blood drift to the placenta (food deliver even as within the uterus). This reasons a scarcity of oxygen and nutrients to the fetus.

Toxic byproducts are produced whilst the frame processes alcohol. Those can then pay attention in the infant's thoughts cells and motive damage.

Damage from alcohol can happen at any point during pregnancy. The beginning of fetal development is the maximum vital for the complete frame, but organs similar to the mind keep to expand during pregnancy. It's impossible to precisely pinpoint all of the development throughout being pregnant, making it unstable to drink alcohol at any time previous to beginning.

It's additionally advocated that you keep away from liquids containing alcohol at the same time as you're seeking to turn out to be pregnant. Many humans don't realise they're pregnant for the primary few weeks of pregnancy (four to 6 weeks). That is as it takes time in your frame to accumulate sufficient hCG (human chorionic gonadotropin, a hormone that develops in early pregnancy) to be detected on a being pregnant check. At some level inside the ones early weeks of being pregnant, the fetus is going thru a big surge of improvement. Alcohol use at some point of this time ought to negatively effect the baby.

How plenty alcohol motives fetal alcohol syndrome?

Any quantity of alcohol during pregnancy can cause fetal alcohol syndrome. There's no secure amount that may be ate up. Damage for your growing infant can appear at any point throughout pregnancy. Even having a drink at the very beginning isn't secure. All alcohol, which include beer, wine, ciders and tough liquor can all reason FAS.

Fetal Alcohol Syndrome diagnosis

There can be no lab test that can show a infant has fetal alcohol syndrome. A lot of its signs and symptoms can look like ADHD.

To diagnose fetal alcohol syndrome, clinical doctors search for unusual facial abilities, decrease-than-common height and weight, small head size, issues with hobby and hyperactivity, and terrible coordination. They also attempt to discover whether or not the mother drank even as they have been pregnant and if so, how plenty.

The signs of fetal alcohol syndrome cannot be cured, but early prognosis and treatment can beautify a little one's improvement and outlook. Research suggests that kids do better once they:

Are recognized earlier than age 6

Are in a loving, nurturing, and solid home at some point of their school years

Aren't exposed to violence

Get precise schooling and social services

Whilst to peer a physician

If you're pregnant and cannot forestall eating, ask your obstetrician, primary care clinical doctor or intellectual fitness professional for help.

Because of the fact early analysis may

additionally additionally help reduce the hazard of prolonged-term issues for kids with fetal alcohol syndrome, allow your little one's physician comprehend if you drank alcohol whilst you were pregnant. Do now not watch for troubles to rise up earlier than trying to find help.

If you have followed a infant or are supplying foster care, you can not recognize if the natural mom drank alcohol at the same time as pregnant — and it can no longer initially occur to you that your infant may also additionally have fetal alcohol syndrome. However, in case your baby has troubles with analyzing and conduct, speak together with his or her doctor so that the underlying motive might be diagnosed.

How is fetal alcohol syndrome (FAS) treated?

Fetal alcohol syndrome isn't curable, and the symptoms will impact your child at some point of lifestyles. However, early treatment of a few signs and signs can reduce the severity and improve your toddler's improvement.

Remedy alternatives can encompass:

Using medicinal tablets to cope with some signs like attention and conduct troubles.

Present process conduct and schooling remedy for emotional and studying worries.

Training you as a determine to super help your infant.

Parental schooling is meant to help parents to assist families address behavioral, academic and social challenges. Mother and father may additionally examine wonderful workouts and tips that may assist their infant adapt to extraordinary situations. Regularly, having a stable and supportive home can assist youngsters with FAS keep away from developing highbrow and emotional problems as they become older.

There also are sure "protective elements" that assist lessen the terrible effect of FAS on a child. These elements can encompass:

Analysis in advance than age 6.

A loving, supportive, solid domestic environment during the college years.

Absence of violence inside the toddler's lifestyles.

Use of particular schooling and social services.

Is there a remedy for fetal alcohol syndrome (FAS)?

There's no treatment for fetal alcohol syndrome. Kids born with this syndrome experience the signs and symptoms and symptoms in some unspecified time in the future of their whole lives. A few signs and symptoms may be managed with treatment via a healthcare enterprise, however they received't leave.

What may be predicted after treatment for fetal alcohol syndrome (FAS)?

No one particular treatment is accurate for absolutely everyone with fetal alcohol syndrome. FAS exists on a spectrum of troubles and the way actually all and sundry is impacted by way of manner of the state of affairs can range significantly. For a few, it's quality to expose their little one's progress within the direction of life, so it's important to have a healthcare issuer you believe.

Complications

Hassle behaviors no longer present at start that may stop result from having fetal alcohol syndrome (secondary disabilities) can also additionally consist of:

Hobby deficit/hyperactivity disorder (ADHD)

Aggression, irrelevant social behavior, and

breaking guidelines and felony hints

Alcohol or drug misuse

Highbrow health troubles, which incorporates melancholy, anxiety or eating problems

Issues staying in or finishing school

Issues with independent residing and with employment

Inappropriate sexual behaviors

Early death through coincidence, homicide or suicide

Prevention

Specialists realise that fetal alcohol syndrome is completely preventable if girls do now not drink alcohol in any respect during being pregnant.

These hints can help prevent fetal alcohol syndrome:

Do no longer drink alcohol in case you're looking to get pregnant. When you have not already stopped ingesting, save you as speedy as you recognize you're pregnant or in case you even think you is probably pregnant. It is in no way too late to save you drinking all through your being pregnant, but the earlier you stop, the higher it's miles for your little one.

Maintain to keep away from alcohol at some stage in your pregnancy. Fetal alcohol syndrome is genuinely preventable in kids whose moms do now not drink at some point of being pregnant.

Undergo in thoughts giving up alcohol in the course of your childbearing years in case you're sexually energetic and you're having unprotected sex. Many pregnancies are unplanned, and damage can get up inside the earliest weeks of pregnancy.

If you have an alcohol trouble, get help before you get pregnant. Get professional help to decide your diploma of dependence on alcohol and to increase a treatment plan.

Does fetal alcohol syndrome (FAS) final into maturity?

Fetal alcohol syndrome in no way is going away. The symptoms of this condition may be with the individual during their entire existence. Through the years, some of secondary effects can appear in people with

FAS, in particular in folks who aren't treated for the situation in early life. The ones are known as secondary outcomes due to the truth they're not part of FAS itself. As a substitute, those secondary effects manifest because of having FAS.

Feasible secondary outcomes of FAS that humans can also revel in into adulthood can embody:

Experiencing intellectual health troubles.

Getting into hassle in university or with the regulation.

Spending time in a highbrow-hospital, a substance abuse treatment middle or prison.

Acting out in sexually inappropriate approaches.

Having difficulty residing on one's personal.

Experiencing unemployment or problem keeping a process.

Receiving remedy as speedy as possible in adolescence can help decrease the chance of growing the ones secondary effects in lifestyles.

CONCLUSION

Alcohol use all through being pregnant reasons existence-lengthy issues that may be very excessive. In case you've fed on alcohol in the course of being pregnant, speak on your healthcare provider. It's critical to make an early evaluation of fetal alcohol syndrome. If you're currently pregnant and ingesting alcohol, prevent straight away to try to decrease the chance of FAS. Communicate in your healthcare organisation to get assist.

THE END